WEIGHT TRAINING WORKOUTS
that
WORK

JAMES ORVIS

Ideal Publishing
Crosslake, Minnesota
weighttrainingworkouts.com

Note to Readers:
The information in this book is intended to provide a safe, effective weight training program. Before starting this or any exercise program please consult with your health care provider. The author and publisher are not responsible for any outcomes.

Weight Training Workouts that Work

Published by:
Ideal Publishing
33806 Pine View Lane
Crosslake, MN 56442

ISBN: 0-9675188-2-2

Layout & Editing: Dusty Rafter and Kay Johnson
Cover Design and Illustrations: Kelley Stafne
Thanks to Lifetime Fitness for the use of their facilities.

Printed in the United States of America
Fourth Printing: February 2004

Library of Congress Catalog Card Number: 99-091355

Contents

Part I: Weight Training Made Easy

Contents

Part II: Exercise Technique Made Easy

Contents

Part II: Continued

Back

Biceps

Triceps

If you have no time to exercise, you'd better reserve a lot of time for disease.

- Dr. Michael Colgan

Weight Training Solves a Major Problem For Being Overweight!

less muscle→burn fewer calories→become fat

Your muscles burn most of the calories and fat you use each and every day. After the age of 20 you are naturally losing muscle unless you include a proper weight training program. You simply need your lean muscles back!

Weight Training Workouts That Work

❑ Take this manual along to your workouts. It is fully illustrated with 12 weeks of proven routines and a simple method to follow and record your progress. No more guesswork.

❑ It shows you exactly how to increase your lean muscle tissue and burn fat at every workout.

❑ No more feeling lost and intimidated when lifting weights.

❑ It is written in easy terms. You can learn weight training today, the right way!

When you sell a man a book you don't sell him just twelve ounces of paper and ink and glue — you sell him a whole new life.

- Christopher Morley

The Four Keys to Weight Training Success

For fast results in weight training you need:

1. Proper form
2. Intensity
3. Variety
4. Consistency

1. Proper Form

The exercises you will perform are described with simple instructions and pictures. Study and practice the exercises with light weights until you become comfortable with the movements. Your form is crucial for maximum results and safety. Follow the exercise technique section as close as possible. Do not watch other people workout, most are doing it wrong.

2. Intensity

Once you learn proper exercise form, you should put total concentration into every rep of each set. Focus on the muscles you are working (study the exercise technique section, so you know which body parts are targeted). Weight Training is 50 percent mental. Learn to concentrate on the muscles you are working, and they will become lean and fat free!

The second part to intensity, and this is very, very important: do as many repetitions as you can, and then try 2 more (always with good form, of course). This is called muscle fatigue. The main reason your body is going to change (lose fat, firm up, become stronger and healthier), is because your body believes it has to in order to survive. It is that simple. If you do not challenge your body by trying a couple more reps, it will stay the same. These are called the "magic reps". They truly are because they will give you a firm and healthy body.

3. Variety

The third big key to lifting weights is variety. Your body needs to be challenged, as in trying two more reps, but it also is super-adaptable. If you do the same workout, day after day, week after week, you will get diminishing returns with every workout - little or no results! Even if you are giving your best effort this will happen. Your body learns very quickly the exercises, weights used, reps, sets, etc. Because it adapts it will use less muscle to perform the exercises. This is exactly what you do not want to happen. You want to keep your body guessing, so it is constantly changing and improving.

4. Consistency

The last key to success is that your body needs regular weight training exercise to make improvements in your health and physical appearance. This does not mean you need to workout for hours every day. This is exactly what you do not want to do (like many people who start an exercise program). You will most likely wear out your body and quit. Consistency means following this manual as close as possible. The proven routines will give you maximum results with a commitment of only a couple hours per week. It's not much time to invest in your health and looks – and it works, too!

Getting Started
What you really need to know!

Barbell (BB)
Long bar usually 4 to 7 feet in length, you hold it with both hands.

Dumbbell (DB)
Short bars about a foot in length, you can hold one in each hand.

Repetition (Rep)
Lifting the weight and lowering the weight to the starting point equals one rep.

Set
Completing as many repetitions as you can on an exercise equals one set.

Tempo
The speed that you lift and lower the weight.
→ **Lift the weight for 1-2 seconds.**
→ **Lower the weight for 2-3 seconds**.
A slow, controlled tempo makes your muscles do all the work (the purpose of lifting weights).
A controlled speed is also easy on your joints.

Breathing
Proper breathing is very important and you need to practice and exaggerate your breathing when you first start weight training. Do not hold your breath!
→ **Exhale when you lift the weight.**
→ **Inhale when you lower the weight.**

Warming up

Always warm-up before weight training. The best way is to do approximately five to ten minutes of a cardiovascular activity. Walking, biking or the stair climber will work nicely. Second, lift light weights, using about half of the weight you will be using during your workout routine. Warm up on all the exercises you are going to perform in your workout. To function properly, your muscles need the increased blood flow that a warm-up provides. When you are ready to give maximum effort, begin your workout routine.

Amount of weight to use on each exercise

Each exercise has a range of weight to choose from in pounds.

→ **The weight is recommended for females.**
→ **Men should double the recommended weight.**

Start with the lightest weight suggested!

These are only recommended weights so you will know where to begin on each exercise. Increase the weights as needed. Your strength will increase substantially within four to six weeks.

Muscle Fibers

Your body is composed of many different kinds of muscle fibers. The two main types we are concerned with are:

1. **Endurance Muscle Fibers**
   They increase in endurance but do not gain much in size or strength. This increase will not assist in burning more calories and fat at rest. Endurance muscles respond best to aerobic activity and high repetition weight training (more than 20 reps).

2. Strength Muscle Fibers

Become stronger, larger and more abundant with proper weight training. This correlates into more calories burned at rest (when you are sitting on the couch!). These are the muscle fibers you want to target when lifting weights. They respond best to 6-15 repetitions to fatigue.

Muscle Fatigue

You cannot complete one more rep with good form.

Rest Periods

Amount of time you rest between sets.

Spotting

A spotter helps the lifter during the exercise. He or she assists in moving the weights into the starting position, helps during the lift so more reps are possible and encourages the lifter to give his or her best effort. A spotter is not necessary on most exercises, but makes lifting weights a safer more productive activity. The most important reason for having a spotter is to be able to complete the last couple of reps to muscle fatigue with proper form.

If exercise equipment is not available

Substitute an available exercise that targets the same muscles from *Part II: Exercise Technique Made Easy*.

Do or do not. There is no try.

- Yoda

Week 1: Basic Exercises

The goal of the first week of weight training is for you to become comfortable with lifting weights. Your body and mind will find it unfamiliar and challenging. Make sure you ease into lifting weights and use proper form. You will love the way the workouts make you feel mentally and physically.

You will be learning seven basic exercises this week. These excellent, safe exercises will work all the major muscle groups in your body. Concentrate on using perfect form. Make sure you are breathing correctly. Remember not to hold your breath!

Keep your muscles tight (flexed) throughout the movements. **Remember on every repetition: 1-2 seconds to lift the weight, 2-3 seconds to lower the weight.** Keep in mind a slow tempo is the best way to lift weights. This is very, very important! Do not copy the way other people workout.

Week 1

☐ Workouts: three non-consecutive days.
   (Example: Monday, Wednesday & Friday)
☐ Two sets per exercise.
☐ 15 repetitions per exercise. Choose from the recommended weight where 15 reps are moderately challenging to complete. You will need to experiment on the weight you use in the beginning. Start with the lightest weight recommended and add more when it becomes too easy.
☐ Men <u>double</u> the recommended starting weight.
☐ Rest 1-2 minutes between sets.
☐ Total body workouts (working all the major muscle groups in your body).

Lets get started on your new body!

Total Body

Workout 1

Exercise	Rep (Goal)	x	Rec. Weight	Set 1		Rest ↑	Set 2	
Dumbbell Bench Press	15	x	5-15		x			x
Lat Pulldown (wide grip)	15	x	30-60		x			x
Leg Press	15	x	50-100		x	1-2 minutes		x
Dumbbell Pullovers	15	x	10-20		x			x
Barbell Curls	15	x	10-20		x			x
Dumbbell Shoulder Press	15	x	3-10		x			x
Crunches	15	x	0		x			x

Notes:

Week 1

Total Body

Workout 2

Exercise	Rep (Goal)	x	Rec. Weight	Set 1		Rest ↑	Set 2	
Dumbbell Bench Press	15	x	5-15		x			x
Lat Pulldown (wide grip)	15	x	30-60		x			x
Leg Press	15	x	50-100		x	1-2 minutes		x
Dumbbell Pullovers	15	x	10-20		x			x
Barbell Curls	15	x	10-20		x			x
Dumbbell Shoulder Press	15	x	3-10		x			x
Crunches	15	x	0		x			x

Notes:

Total Body

Workout 3

Exercise	Rep (Goal)	x	Rec. Weight	Set 1		Rest ↑	Set 2	
Dumbbell Bench Press	15	x	5-15		x			x
Lat Pulldown (wide grip)	15	x	30-60		x			x
Leg Press	15	x	50-100		x			x
Dumbbell Pullovers	15	x	10-20		x	1-2 minutes		x
Barbell Curls	15	x	10-20		x			x
Dumbbell Shoulder Press	15	x	3-10		x			x
Crunches	15	x	0		x			x

Notes:

"I knew nothing about weightlifting when I started, only what I had seen on TV and at the gym…but loving exercise, I thought I'd give the program a try. In the short time I have been lifting, I have seen results that have astonished me. My upper body, besides being much stronger now, has <u>form</u> and keeps on improving. The overall strength and workout to my full body is making a big difference in how I feel and how I perceive myself. Weight training for overall fitness is much more <u>fun</u> and exciting than I ever thought and I will be continuing with the program."

- Chris B., age 45

Week 2: Challenging Reps

How was the first week? Feels great doesn't it?! You are on your way to a firmer and healthier body!

Did you know that being overweight is your greatest health risk? Body fat causes more illness than all environmental and nutritional problems, more than smoking, alcohol, and all other drugs put together[1].

"Your Health Is Your Wealth"

Weight training is the first and most important step in being healthy and fit, because it brings back your youthful muscles.

Week 2

- Workouts: three non-consecutive days.
- Continue working with the same seven exercises.
- Two sets per exercise.
- 15 reps per exercise but the last 2 reps should be more challenging this week. So increase the weights when needed.
- Rest 1-2 minutes between sets.
- Total body workouts.

[1]Colgan, Michael. The New Nutrition. C.I. Publications, 1994.

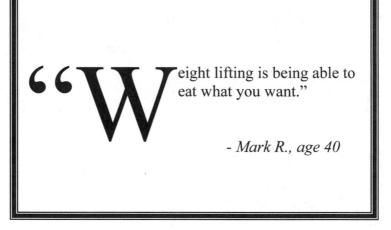

"**W**eight lifting is being able to eat what you want."

- Mark R., age 40

Men are born to succeed, not to fail.

- Henry David Thoreau

Week 2

Challenging Reps

Total Body

Workout 1

Exercise	Rep (Goal)	x	Rec. Weight	Set 1	Rest ↑	Set 2
Dumbbell Bench Press	15	x	5-15	x		x
Lat Pulldown (wide grip)	15	x	30-60	x		x
Leg Press	15	x	50-100	x		x
Dumbbell Pullovers	15	x	10-20	x		x
Barbell Curls	15	x	10-20	x		x
Dumbbell Shoulder Press	15	x	3-10	x		x
Crunches	15	x	0	x		x

1-2 minutes (Rest)

Notes:

Total Body

Workout 2

Exercise	Rep (Goal)	x	Rec. Weight	Set 1		Rest ↑	Set 2	
Dumbbell Bench Press	15	✗	5-15		✗		✗	
Lat Pulldown (wide grip)	15	✗	30-60		✗		✗	
Leg Press	15	✗	50-100		✗	1-2 minutes	✗	
Dumbbell Pullovers	15	✗	10-20		✗		✗	
Barbell Curls	15	✗	10-20		✗		✗	
Dumbbell Shoulder Press	15	✗	3-10		✗		✗	
Crunches	15	✗	0				✗	

Notes:

Week 2

Challenging Reps

Total Body

Workout 3

Exercise	Rep (Goal)	x	Rec. Weight	Set 1		Rest ↑	Set 2	
Dumbbell Bench Press	15	x	5-15		x			x
Lat Pulldown (wide grip)	15	x	30-60		x			x
Leg Press	15	x	50-100		x	1-2 minutes		x
Dumbbell Pullovers	15	x	10-20		x			x
Barbell Curls	15	x	10-20		x			x
Dumbbell Shoulder Press	15	x	3-10		x			x
Crunches	15	x	0		x			x

Notes:

Week 3: Adding New Exercises

Are you feeling firmer? Stronger? Can you start to feel muscles you never knew existed? This is exciting stuff! You are changing your body permanently – reversing the aging process. Keep it up!

This is one of the most important points of the manual. **Your body changes (adds lean muscle tissue, loses fat) because it believes it has to in order to survive.** How is this accomplished? One way is to lift a weight that your body is not accustomed to lifting. The last couple of reps that are challenging with perfect form are the "magic reps". They signal your body that you could not lift the weight. To be able to lift the weight next time, your body will add lean muscle tissue. This burns a tremendous amount of calories 24 hours a day because your body is repairing and building the muscle and maintaining it (muscles need a constant supply of calories to keep it alive). Pretty simple. And simple answers are always the best!

Week 3

- ❑ Workouts: three non-consecutive days.
- ❑ During week 3 you are going to add new exercises.
- ❑ On new exercises: 2 sets for 15 reps and make the last 2 reps challenging.
- ❑ On the exercises you have been performing the first two weeks, do 2 sets each for 12 repetitions that are challenging. Increase the weights when needed.
- ❑ Rest 1-2 minutes between sets.
- ❑ Total body workouts.

"**W**hy do I weight train? I love feeling fit! Regular workouts give me many positive benefits: increased self-esteem, lower stress and most importantly, it gives me the energy to be active and enjoy life. Weight training is essential to feeling and looking great!!"

- Dusty R., age 26

Adding New Exercises

Total Body

Workout 1

Exercise	Rep (Goal)	x	Rec. Weight	Set 1		Rest ↑	Set 2	
Lat Pulldown (triangle bar)	12	x	40-70		x			x
Tricep Pushdowns	15	x	15-30		x	1-2 minutes		x
Leg Extensions	15	x	20-50		x			x
Leg Curls	15	x	20-50		x			x
Dumbbell Shoulder Press	12	x	5-15		x			x
Ab Bench Crunches	15	x	0		x			x

Notes:

Total Body

Workout 2

Exercise	Rep (Goal)	x	Rec. Weight	Set 1		Rest ↑	Set 2	
Dumbbell Curls	15	x	5-15		x			x
Side Lateral Raises	15	x	1-8		x			x
Dumbbell Bench Press	15	x	5-15		x	1-2 minutes		x
Calf Raises	15	x	50-100		x			x
Leg Extensions	15	x	20-50		x			x
Leg Curls	15	x	20-50		x			x
Ab Bench Crunches	15		0					

Notes:

Total Body

Workout 3

Exercise	Rep (Goal)	x	Rec. Weight	Set 1		Rest ↑	Set 2	
Leg Press	12	x	50-100		x			x
Dumbbell Curls	12	x	5-15		x			x
Lunges (right leg)	15	x	0		x			x
Lunges (left leg)	15	x	0		x			x
Tricep Pushdowns	12	x	15-30		x	1-2 minutes		x
Side Lateral Raises	15	x	1-8		x			x
Ab Bench Crunches	15	x	0		x			x

Notes:

You gain strength, courage and confidence by every experience in which you really stop to look fear in the face. You are able to say to yourself, "I lived through this horror. I can take the next thing that comes along."

You must do the thing you think you cannot do.

- Eleanor Roosevelt

Week 4: All Exercises to Fatigue

Wow, the fourth week is already here! Are you being consistent with your workouts?

As the saying goes, "80 percent of success is showing up." It is so very true with weight training. Your muscles become stronger and firmer when they are worked 1 to 3 times per week. They become smaller and softer (and burn fewer calories) when you are not consistent with your workout schedule. A couple hours per week to have the body you desire. **Lifting weights is the fat burning pill you have been looking for all these years!**

Here is what to do if you do not feel like lifting weights today. Go to your workout and try it for ten minutes, and then make a decision. You will almost always keep on going because it feels fantastic and you are looking and feeling better every day. Try it – it works!

What you really want to concentrate on in week four is fatiguing your muscles in the 10 to 12 rep range for most exercises (unless otherwise specified). You will get maximum lean muscle tissue and fat loss when you hit muscle fatigue around 10-12 reps.

Two important points about 10 repetitions to fatigue.

1. In the 10-rep range, the first rep feels heavy. This will feel different. If the first rep feels light, you can do 20, 30, 40 reps or more. Your muscle size, strength and fat burning ability does <u>not</u> improve a great deal when you are able to complete more than 20 reps. Remember, those are endurance muscle fibers. You build more endurance (which is good), but not your main goal with weight training.

2. Your muscles do not count, they respond to a stress. Do not do 10 reps and stop if you can do more. *"I did 10 reps and now my body is going to be lean and fit."* No, do as many reps as you can with good form and increase the weights next time if it was too light. Your goal is to hit muscle fatigue around 10 repetitions. Make every set your best and you will see the fantastic changes!

You will continue to add new exercises this week. Don't forget to study how each exercise is performed and concentrate on which muscles are being targeted.

Week 4
- ❑ Workouts: three non-consecutive days.
- ❑ Continue to add new exercises.
- ❑ <u>Three sets</u> per exercise.
- ❑ 10-12 repetitions to fatigue on most exercise.
- ❑ Rest 1 to 2 minutes between sets.
- ❑ Total body workouts.

"**W**eight training is simply a way of life for me. I thoroughly enjoy it. Even though I'm getting older, I feel <u>younger</u>. My self-esteem has increased and I have more energy, which means more quality time with my kids. I have learned what dedication and discipline really mean and that in itself makes me feel great in all aspects of my life."

- Scott J., age 30

Total Body

Workout 1

Exercise	Rep (Goal)	x	Rec. Weight	Set 1			Rest ↑	Set 2			Rest ↑	Set 3		
Dumbbell Squats	15	x	5-15			x	1-2 minutes			x	1-2 minutes			x
Dumbbell Rows (right arm)	15	x	10-20			x				x				x
Dumbbell Rows (left arm)	15	x	10-20			x				x				x
Barbell Curls	10	x	15-25			x				x				x
Ab Bench Crunches	15	x	0			x				x				x
Crunches	15	x	0			x				x				x

Notes:

All Exercises to Fatigue

Total Body

Workout 2

Exercise	Rep (Goal)	x	Rec. Weight	Set 1		Rest ↑	Set 2		Rest ↑	Set 3	
Lat Pulldown (underhand)	12	x	40-70		x			x			x
Deadlifts	15	x	0-45		x	1-2 minutes		x	1-2 minutes		x
Leg Curls	15	x	30-60		x			x			x
Calf Raises	15	x	50-100		x			x			x
Barbell Shoulder Press	15	x	15-40		x			x			x

Notes:

Week 4

All Exercises to Fatigue

Total Body

Workout 3

Exercise	Rep (Goal)	x	Rec. Weight	Set 1		Rest → 1-2 minutes	Set 2		Rest → 1-2 minutes	Set 3	
Leg Extensions	12	x	30-60		x			x			x
Barbell Squats	15	x	25-50		x			x			x
Incline DB Bench Press	12	x	10-20		x			x			x
Dumbbell Flys	15	x	3-10		x			x			x
Dumbbell Curls	10	x	5-15		x			x			x
Reverse Crunches	10	x	0		x			x			x

Notes:

Week 5: Super Sets

This is where the workouts become really fun! You are seeing results, feeling better and healthier and your body is thriving on the workouts. Remember, the four big keys are:

1. Proper form
2. Intensity
3. Consistency
4. Variety

In the fifth week we will tackle the problem of variety in your workouts. Your body is super-adaptable, which means it is good at staying the same, even when you want it to change (lose fat, build muscle). You need to trick it into changing and one important way is to add variety to your workouts.

Your body can adapt to a certain training routine in approximately 2 weeks. This means you will get little or no results if you do the same workout longer than 2 weeks in a row. The same exercises, same weight, same order, same rest periods between sets, etc.

Weight Training Workouts that Work is designed with 2 weeks of proven workout routines and then switches to a completely different routine for the next 2 weeks. This keeps your body always guessing and changing, which is exactly what you want it to do.

In the fifth week you will learn Super Sets, a great way to change your body.

Super Sets

1. Perform one set of the first exercise (exercise a).
2. Immediately perform a set of the second exercise (exercise b).

Example: a) Dumbbell Pullover
↓ no rest
b) Lat Pulldown

The two exercises should be as close together as possible (in proximity), so you can do them back to back with as little rest in between as possible.

Week 5

□ Workouts: three non-consecutive days.
□ Three Super Sets per exercises.
□ 10-15 repetitions to fatigue (remember to increase the weights when they are to light).
□ Rest 1-2 minutes after each Super Set. No rest during the Super Set!
□ Total body workouts.

"When I turned 27, I noticed significant fluctuations in my weight. I was always told my metabolism would catch up to me. IT DID! I felt I needed to do something before my weight and tone of my muscles got away from me. Working out has afforded me the ability to continue to cat what I want with little effort to maintain my weight and shape. My energy level is high and I look better than ever!"

- Traci O., age 28

Week 5

Super Sets

Total Body

Workout 1

Exercise	Rep (Goal)	×	Rec. Weight	Set 1		Rest →	Set 2		Rest →	Set 3	
a) Leg Extensions	15	×	30-60		×			×			×
b) Leg Press	15	×	50-100		×			×			×
No Rest											
a) Dumbbell Pullovers	12	×	10-20		×			×			×
b) Lat Pulldown (triangle bar)	12	×	40-70		×			×			×
No Rest											
a)Dumbbell Flys	12	×	3-10		×			×			×
b) Dumbbell Bench Press	12	×	5-15		×			×			×
No Rest											
a) Crunches	15	×	0		×			×			×
b) Ab Bench Crunches	15	×	0		×			×			×

Rest → **1-2 minutes** (between Set 1 and Set 2)

Rest → **1-2 minutes** (between Set 2 and Set 3)

Notes:

Week 5

Super Sets

Total Body

Workout 2

Rest →	Exercise	Rep (Goal)	×	Rec. Weight	Set 1		Rest ↑	Set 2		Rest ↑	Set 3	
	a) Deadlifts	15	×	20-45		×			×			×
No Rest	b) Leg Curls	15	×	30-60		×	1-2 minutes		×	1-2 minutes		×
	a) Dumbbell Shoulder Press	10	×	5-15		×			×			×
No Rest	b) Side Lateral Raises	10	×	3-10		×			×			×
	a) Barbell Curls	10	×	15-30		×			×			×
No Rest	b) Lat Pulldown (underhand)	10	×	40-70		×			×			×
	a) Reverse Crunches	10	×	0		×			×			×
No Rest	b) Ab Bench Crunches	15	×	0		×			×			×

Notes:

Week 5

Super Sets

Total Body

Workout 3

Rest →	Exercise	Rep (Goal)	x	Rec. Weight	Set 1		Rest ↑	Set 2		Rest ↑	Set 3	
No Rest	a) Leg Curls	15	x	40-70		x			x			x
	b) Leg Press	15	x	75-150		x			x			x
No Rest	a) Dumbbell Pullovers	10	x	15-30		x	1-2 minutes		x	1-2 minutes		x
	b) Lat Pulldown (wide grip)	10	x	40-70		x			x			x
No Rest	a) Barbell Squats	15	x	30-60		x			x			x
	b) Leg Extensions	15	x	30-60		x			x			x
No Rest	a) Crunches	15	x	0		x			x			x
	b) Ab Bench Crunches	15	x	0		x			x			x

Notes:

Week 6: Super Sets

Now that you have completed 15 workouts, are you seeing the physical results of your commitment to a better body? Fifteen workouts is the magic point where your body really starts to change.

- Fat loss
- Firm muscles you never knew existed
- Increase in strength and energy
- Body shape changes
- Loose and better fitting clothes

These Are the Permanent Results You Wanted!

In the sixth week, you will complete one more week of Super Sets. You will add two variations to your workout routines to keep you body improving. Up to this point, you have been doing total body workouts. Now you will occasionally emphasize different body parts in each workout, called split routines. Example: legs on Mondays, upper body on Wednesdays, etc. This lets your body concentrate and improve on a specific area and lets non-worked muscles rest and recover for their next workout.

Also, sometimes you should lift weights on two consecutive days to stimulate results. Your body becomes used to lifting weights on the same days, with the same time off between workouts. Training on consecutive days (every couple of weeks) will solve this problem.

Week 6

- ❑ Three workouts.
- ❑ Workouts 1 and 2 on consecutive days.
- ❑ Workout 3 on a non-consecutive day. (Example: Monday - Tuesday - Friday)
- ❑ Three Super Sets per exercise.
- ❑ Rest 1 to 2 minutes <u>after each Super Set</u>. No rest during the Super Set!
- ❑ 10-12 reps to fatigue.
- ❑ Split routines.

"I did aerobics up to 90 minutes a day, 6 days per week and I was getting nowhere. Weightlifting changed all that. Now my workouts are no longer than 45 minutes, the variety of exercises is practically endless, and best of all, I SEE RESULTS! Weightlifting is a sure-fire way to change the shape of your body. There is no question that cardiovascular workouts are great for the heart and lungs and bolster your mood. But if you want to burn calories more efficiently, improve your strength and flexibility, and noticeably alter the way you look, pump some iron!

- Beth W., age 43

Week 6

Super Sets

Legs and Abs

Workout 1

Exercise	Rep (Goal)	x	Rec. Weight	Set 1		Rest →	Set 2		Rest →	Set 3	
a) Leg Extensions	12	x	40-70		x			x			x
b) Leg Press	12	x	75-150		x			x			x
a) Deadlifts	15	x	20-45		x	1-2 minutes		x	1-2 minutes		x
b) Leg Curls	10	x	30-60		x			x			x
a) Reverse Crunches	10	x	0		x			x			x
b) Ab Bench Crunches	12	x	0		x			x			x

No Rest   No Rest   No Rest

Rest ↓

Notes:

Chest, Shoulders, and Triceps

Workout 2

Rest →	Exercise	Rep (Goal)	x	Rec. Weight	Set 1	Rest ↑	Set 2	Rest ↑	Set 3
	a) Dumbbell Flys	10	x	5-15	x		x		x
No Rest	b) Dumbbell Bench Press	10	x	10-20	x	1-2 minutes	x	1-2 minutes	x
	a) Barbell Bench Press	10	x	30-60	x		x		x
No Rest	b) Tricep Pushdowns	10	x	15-30	x		x		x
	a) Barbell Shoulder Press	10	x	20-40	x		x		x
No Rest	b) Side Lateral Raises	10	x	3-10	x		x		x

Notes:

Week 6

Super Sets

Abs, Back, and Biceps

Workout 3

Rest →	Exercise	Rep (Goal)	×	Rec. Weight	Set 1		Rest ↑	Set 2		Rest ↑	Set 3	
No Rest	a) Reverse Crunches	10	×	0		×			×			×
	b) Ab Bench Crunches	15	×	0		×			×			×
No Rest	a) Dumbbell Pullovers	10	×	15-30		×	1-2 minutes		×	1-2 minutes		×
	b) Lat Pulldown (wide grip)	10	×	40-70		×			×			×
No Rest	a) Dumbbell Pullovers	12	×	10-20		×			×			×
	b) Lat Pulldown (underhand)	12	×	30-60		×			×			×
No Rest	a) Dumbbell Curls	12	×	5-15		×			×			×
	b) Barbell Curls	12	×	15-30		×			×			×

Notes:

Week 7: Drop Sets

Is your strength increasing? You should be considerably stronger by the seventh week. If you are not becoming stronger, make sure you are increasing the weight so the last 2 reps are challenging in the appropriate rep range. Make it a personal goal to try one more repetition on each exercise. By week seven completing one more rep than you thought possible is an inspiring feeling. Your body and mind will thrive on it and make you feel years younger. It is one of the best investments you can make for your health.

In the seventh and eighth weeks you will do Drop Sets, another great method for more results.

Drop Sets

1. Do a set of an exercise to fatigue.
2. Immediately lower the weight and go to fatigue on the same exercise for the second time.
3. Lower the weight again (with no rest) for the third and final set to fatigue.

Tip: Drop Sets are most effective with a spotter so they can change the weight for you.

Tip: The amount of weight you lower on each set will vary. Approximately a 30 percent drop on each set is the most effective. Each exercise and individual is different. You will have to experiment in the beginning to discover what works best for you.

Example: Leg Press

SET 1A): 100 lbs. X 12 reps
↓ no rest

SET 1B): 70 lbs. X 12 reps
↓ no rest

SET 1C): 50 lbs. X 12 reps
Drop Set is complete
↓ Rest 2-3 minutes
Go to the next exercise

Week 7

- ❑ Workouts: three non-consecutive days.
- ❑ Drop Sets: 1 per exercise.
- ❑ Reps: 10-15 to fatigue.
- ❑ Rest 2-3 minutes after <u>each Drop Set is complete</u>. No rest during the Drop Set.
- ❑ Split routines.
- ❑ Remember to lower the weight about 30 percent each drop.

"**I** lift weights to lose fat without dieting."

- Bonnie J., age 45

Week 7

Drop Sets

Legs and Abs

Workout 1

Exercise	Rep (Goal)	x	Rec. Weight	Set 1a	Rest ↑	Set 1b	Rest ↑	Set 1c
Leg Extensions	15-15-15	x	40-70	x		x		x
Leg Curls	10-10-10	x	40-70	x		x		x
Calf Raises	15-15-15	x	75-125	x	No Rest	x	No Rest	x
Leg Press	12-12-12	x	75-150	x		x		x
Crunches	15-15-15	x	0-10	x		x		x

Notes:

Upper Body

Workout 2

Exercise	Rep (Goal)	x	Rec. Weight	Set 1a			Rest ↑	Set 1b			Rest ↑	Set 1c		
Dumbbell Rows (right arm)	10-10-10	x	10-25		x		No Rest		x		No Rest		x	
Dumbbell Rows (left arm)	10-10-10	x	10-25		x				x				x	
Lat Pulldown (triangle bar)	10-10-10	x	40-70		x				x				x	
Barbell Bench Press	10-10-10	x	30-60		x				x				x	
Dumbbell Pullovers	10-10-10	x	15-30		x				x				x	
Dumbbell Curls	10-10-10	x	15-30		x				x				x	

Notes:

Week 7

Drop Sets

Legs

Workout 3

Exercise	Rep (Goal)	x	Rec. Weight	Set 1a		Rest ↑	Set 1b		Rest ↑	Set 1c	
Leg Press	12-12-12	x	100-200		x	No Rest		x	No Rest		x
Leg Curls	10-10-10	x	40-70		x			x			x
Leg Extensions	15-15-15	x	30-60		x			x			x
Dumbbell Squats	15-15-15	x	10-25		x			x			x
Calf Raises	15-15-15	x	75-150		x			x			x

Notes:

Week 8: Drop Sets

Do you have a workout partner? One of the best things you can do to insure success in meeting your fitness goals is to find a workout partner. They motivate you when you do not feel like working out. You motivate them when they are feeling a little lazy. It can make exercise a more enjoyable activity, when you can share it with someone else and you can spot for each other. Spotting is especially important when you do those last 2 important reps to muscle fatigue. They will help you complete the last couple of reps in a safe environment and encourage you to use proper form.

You will continue to do Drop Sets during the eighth week. Your body needs a short break (5-7 days) from weight training approximately every two months. This allows your muscles and all the systems of your body to fully recuperate and re-energize. Without a break from lifting every couple of months, you can become overtrained. This leads to a plateau or a loss in results. You will lift weights only one time this week to avoid overtraining. When you come back next week, you will feel energetic and you will not be able to wait to workout again!

Week 8

- Workouts: one (early in the week).
- Drop Sets: 1 per exercise.
- 10-15 reps to fatigue.
- Rest 2-3 minutes after each Drop Set is complete. No rest during the Drop Set.
- Total body workout.
- Lower the weight about 30 percent each drop.

"I have integrated weight training into my everyday life just like brushing my teeth and washing my hair. It is important for me to make the time to workout to maintain the quality of my overall health and well being. Lifting weights contributes as much to my mental health as my physical health. I can feel the impact of missing a week. I am more sensitive to stress and I am tired when I do not weight train."

- Sue W., age 43

Week Eight

Drop Sets

Total Body

Workout 1

Exercise	Rep (Goal)	x	Rec. Weight	Set 1a	Rest ↑	Set 1b	Rest ↑	Set 1c
Barbell Shoulder Press	10-10-10	x	20-40	x		x		x
Leg Extensions	10-10-10	x	40-70	x		x		x
Barbell Squats	15-15-15	x	30-60	x	No Rest	x	No Rest	x
Dumbbell Bench Press	10-10-10	x	10-25	x		x		x
Tricep Pushdowns	10-10-10	x	15-30	x		x		x
Crunches (with weight)	10-10-10	x	0-25	x		x		x

Notes:

Passion is in all great searches and is necessary to all creative endeavors.

- W. Eugene Smith

Week 9: Pyramid-Up

Knowledge is power. The more you know about your body and how it works, the better. Scientific advances are offering us new and more effective ways to build a healthier, more fit body. Every day there is progress in the area of health and fitness. Browse through fitness magazines, books, the Internet, newspapers, etc. This will help you stay motivated and add new information for greater results.

In weeks nine and ten you will use the Pyramid-Up routine.

Pyramid-Up

- ❑ Three sets of an exercise.
- ❑ Increase the weights each set.
- ❑ Lower rep goal each set.
- ❑ 3 minutes rest between sets.

Example: Barbell Bench Press

SET 1: 12 reps x 45 lbs.
↓ Rest 3 minutes
Increase the weights

SET 2: 10 reps x 55 lbs.
↓ Rest 3 minutes
Increase the weights

SET 3: 8 reps x 65 lbs.
↓ Rest 3 minutes
Go to the next exercise

Week 9

- ❑ Workouts: three non-consecutive days.
- ❑ Pyramid-Up: 3 sets per exercise.
- ❑ 8-12 reps to fatigue.
- ❑ Rest 3 minutes between sets.
- ❑ Split routines.

"Since I started strength training, I have noticed more changes in my appearance. Before beginning a weight training workout program, I did a lot of aerobic exercises and did not see any changes. Lifting weights has provided me with better results, which keeps me motivated and looking forward to each workout. I used to think that lifting would make me look masculine and get *too big*. Just the opposite! I have actually made areas shrink due to decreasing the fat and replacing it with lean muscle".

- Shelley E., age 32

Week Nine

Pyramid-Up

Chest, Shoulders, Triceps, and Abs

Workout 1

Exercise	Rep (Goal)	x	Rec. Weight	Set 1			Rest →	Set 2			Rest →	Set 3		
Barbell Bench Press	12-10-8	x	35-75		x				x				x	
Incline DB Bench Press	12-10-8	x	10-25		x				x				x	
Dumbbell Shoulder Press	12-10-8	x	5-15		x		3 minutes		x		3 minutes		x	
Tricep Pushdowns	12-10-8	x	20-40		x				x				x	
Crunches (with weight)	12-10-8	x	5-25		x				x				x	

Notes:

Week Nine

Pyramid-Up

Legs and Abs

Workout 2

Exercise	Rep (Goal)	x	Rec. Weight	Set 1		Rest ↑	Set 2		Rest ↑	Set 3	
Barbell Squats	12-10-8	x	30-75		x			x			x
Leg Press	12-10-8	x	100-200		x	3 minutes		x	3 minutes		x
Leg Extensions	12-10-8	x	40-70		x			x			x
Crunches (with weight)	12-10-8	x	5-25		x			x			x

Notes:

Pyramid-Up

Back, Biceps, and Abs

Workout 3

Exercise	Rep (Goal)	x	Rec. Weight	Set 1		Rest ↑	Set 2		Rest ↑	Set 3	
Dumbbell Pullovers	12-10-8	x	15-30	x			x			x	
Lat Pulldown (underhand)	12-10-8	x	50-100	x		3 minutes	x		3 minutes	x	
Dumbbell Curls	12-10-8	x	10-20	x			x			x	
Barbell Curls	12-10-8	x	20-45	x			x			x	
Reverse Crunches	12-10-8	x	0	x			x			x	

Notes:

Week 10: Pyramid-Up

Losing motivation? It happens to the best of us. Just remember that people who are the happiest and get the most out of life, challenge themselves. Your body is the same way. If it is not challenged consistently, it can become unhealthy and unsightly.

According the Dr. Michael Colgan, one of the leading scientists in health and fitness, 1 out of 10,000 people are genetically overweight. 1 out of 10,000! Let's not blame our parents for our bodies. We all come in different shapes and sizes, but almost everybody can look good and feel great with the proper knowledge and desire!

Strive for small changes in your body every week. This will add up to what you want in a very short time. Making progress in the way you look and feel is a very rewarding experience. People will notice the changes!

Week 10
- Workouts: three non-consecutive days.
- Pyramid-Up: 3 sets per exercise.
- 8-12 reps to fatigue.
- 3 minutes rest between sets.
- Split routines.

"Weight lifting and dedication have really enhanced my life. My all-around energy has improved, and the fat loss and increased strength has stabilized my entire body to the point where my frequent trips to the chiropractor have been eliminated. It hasn't been easy, but what in life is? Go for it!"

- Doug B., age 38

Chest, Shoulders, Triceps, and Abs

Workout 1

Exercise	Rep (Goal)	x	Rec. Weight	Set 1		Rest ↑	Set 2		Rest ↑	Set 3	
Bench Press	12-10-8	x	35-75		x			x			x
Incline DB Bench Press	12-10-8	x	10-25		x	3 minutes		x	3 minutes		x
Dumbbell Shoulder Press	12-10-8	x	5-15		x			x			x
Tricep Pushdowns	12-10-8	x	20-40		x			x			x
Crunches (with weight)	12-10-8	x	5-25		x			x			x

Notes:

Pyramid-Up

Legs

Workout 2

Exercise	Rep (Goal)	x	Rec. Weight	Set 1			Rest ↑	Set 2			Rest ↑	Set 3		
Barbell Squats	12-10-8	x	45-85		x				x				x	
Leg Press	12-10-8	x	100-200		x		3 minutes		x		3 minutes		x	
Leg Extensions	12-10-8	x	40-70		x				x				x	
Calf Raises	12-10-8	x	75-150		x				x				x	

Notes:

Back, Biceps, and Abs

Workout 3

Exercise	Rep (Goal)	x	Rec. Weight	Set 1	Rest ↑	Set 2	Rest ↑	Set 3
Dumbbell Pullovers	12-10-8	x	15-30	x		x		x
Lat Pulldown (triangle bar)	12-10-8	x	50-100	x		x		x
Dumbbell Curls	12-10-8	x	10-20	x		x		x
Barbell Curls	12-10-8	x	20-45	x		x		x
Reverse Crunches	12-10-8	x	0	x		x		x

Rest columns: **3 minutes**, **3 minutes**

Notes:

Far better it is to dare mighty things, to win glorious triumphs even though checkered by failure, than to rank with those poor spirits who neither enjoy nor suffer much because they live in the gray twilight that knows neither victory nor defeat.

- Theodore Roosevelt

Week 11: 3-in-a-Row

Visualize. Are you concentrating and visualizing on the muscles you are working? The mind-body connection is very important for maximum results in weight training. It will become easier and easier to feel your muscles when you become stronger and leaner.

Also, it is more important how you lift the weight than how much weight you lift. Yes, you need to increase the weights when you become stronger, but remember to lift slow with concentration and to visualize the muscles you are working. The goal is to fatigue the muscles with proper form. Go wear out those muscles!

In weeks eleven and twelve you will do the 3-in-a-Row routine, an outstanding fat burner and muscle toner.

3-in-a-Row
- Same exercise.
- Same weight.
- Same rep goal.
- 3 sets.
- 30 seconds rest between the 3 sets.

Example: Barbell Squats

SET 1: 10 reps x 45 lbs.
↓ Rest only 30 seconds

SET 2: 10 reps x 45 lbs.
↓ Rest only 30 seconds

SET 3: 10 reps x 45 lbs.
Set is complete
↓ Rest 3 minutes
Go to the next exercise

Tip: You probably will not be able to reach your rep goal on the second and third set. This is to be expected because of muscle fatigue and the purpose of the 3-in-a Row routine. Just complete as many reps as you can with proper form.

Week 11

- ❑ Workouts: <u>two, non-consecutive days</u>.
- ❑ 3-in-a-Row routine on each exercise.
- ❑ 10 reps to fatigue.
- ❑ 3 minutes rest between <u>exercises</u>. Only 30 seconds rest during 3-in-a-Row routine.
- ❑ Total body workouts.

"I tend to have a lot of back problems. Going to the chiropractor was a regular event in my life. With back problems, I was skeptical at first. After I started weight training, I felt so much more physically fit and my back problems disappeared. It has really made a difference in my life".

- Angela P., age 27

Total Body

Workout 1

Exercise	Rep (Goal)	x	Rec. Weight	Set 1		Rest ↑	Set 2		Rest ↑	Set 3	
Barbell Squats	10	x	45-100	x			x			x	
Lunges (right leg)	10	x	0-20	x		30 seconds	x		30 seconds	x	
Lunges (left leg)	10	x	0-20	x			x			x	
Lat Pulldown (wide grip)	10	x	50-100	x			x			x	
Incline DB Bench Press	10	x	10-25	x			x			x	

Notes:

3-in-a-Row

Total Body

Workout 2

Exercise	Rep (Goal)	x	Rec. Weight	Set 1			Rest →	Set 2			Rest →	Set 3		
Leg Press	10	x	100-200		x				x				x	
Leg Press	10	x	100-200		x				x				x	
Dumbbell Pullovers	10	x	15-30		x				x				x	
Dumbbell Pullovers	10	x	15-30		x				x				x	
Incline DB Bench Press	10	x	10-25		x		30 seconds		x		30 seconds		x	
Incline DB Bench Press	10	x	10-25		x				x				x	
Crunches (with weight)	15	x	0-25		x				x				x	

Notes:

The thing always happens that you really believe in;
and the belief in a thing makes it happen.

- Frank Lloyd Wright

Week 12: 3-in-a-Row

Wow! The last week already! Don't you feel great and love the changes your body has made? Until you start this program, it is hard to explain how great you will look and feel. Keep it up and make weight training an essential part of your life. Tell a friend and show them the great discovery you have made!

Week 12
- ❑ Workouts: <u>Three consecutive days</u>.
- ❑ Continue 3-in-a-Row routine on each exercise.
- ❑ 8-10 reps to fatigue.
- ❑ Rest 3 minutes between exercises. Rest only 30 seconds during 3-in-a-Row routine.
- ❑ Split routines.

"I weight train to increase flexibility and to build the muscle that has atrophied from injury and lack of activity. For approximately the last 10 years, I have experienced chronic lower back pain. <u>After 5 months of lifting weights, I can perform most activities without pain</u>. The more I train, the more confidence I have to push my body further without the fear of injury. I feel like a new person."

- Tom N. age 54

Week 12

Legs and Back

Workout 1

Exercise	Rep (Goal)	x	Rec. Weight	Set 1			Rest →	Set 2			Rest →	Set 3		
Leg Press	10	x	100-200	x				x				x		
Leg Curls	10	x	40-80	x				x				x		
Deadlifts	15	x	20-60	x				x				x		
Lat Pulldown (triangle bar)	8	x	50-100	x				x				x		
Dumbbell Rows (left arm)	8	x	15-30	x			30 seconds	x			30 seconds	x		
Dumbbell Rows (right arm)	8	x	15-30	x				x				x		

Notes:

Week 12

3-in-a-Row

Chest, Shoulders and Arms

Workout 2

Exercise	Rep (Goal)	x	Rec. Weight	Set 1			Rest ↑	Set 2			Rest ↑	Set 3		
Barbell Bench Press	8	x	35-75		✗				✗				✗	
Dumbbell Shoulder Press	8	x	20-45		✗		30 seconds		✗		30 seconds		✗	
Side Lateral Raises	8	x	5-12		✗				✗				✗	
Dumbbell Bench Press	8	x	10-25		✗				✗				✗	
Barbell Curls	8	x	20-45		✗				✗				✗	
Tricep Pushdowns	8	x	20-50		✗				✗				✗	

Notes:

Abs and Legs

Workout 3

Exercise	Rep (Goal)	x	Rec. Weight	Set 1		Rest →	Set 2		Rest →	Set 3	
Ab Bench Crunches	10	x	0		x			x			x
Reverse Crunches	10	x	0		x			x			x
Crunches	10	x	0-25		x			x			x
Lunges (left leg)	10	x	0-20		x	30 seconds		x	30 seconds		x
Lunges (right leg)	10	x	0-20		x			x			x
Leg Press	15	x	75-150		x			x			x

Notes:

Always bear in mind that your own resolution to success is more important than any other one thing.

- Abraham Lincoln

Conclusion: What's next?

After completing *Weight Training Workouts that Work*, go back to week one and start the program over. Try to improve on each exercise by completing 1 more repetition and/or increasing the weight.

After going through the program a second time, you can start to make up your own workouts. Just plug in different exercises to the proven workout routines and find the ones that are the most effective for you.

The real secret of success is enthusiasm.

- Walter Chrysler

Part II
Exercise Technique Made Easy

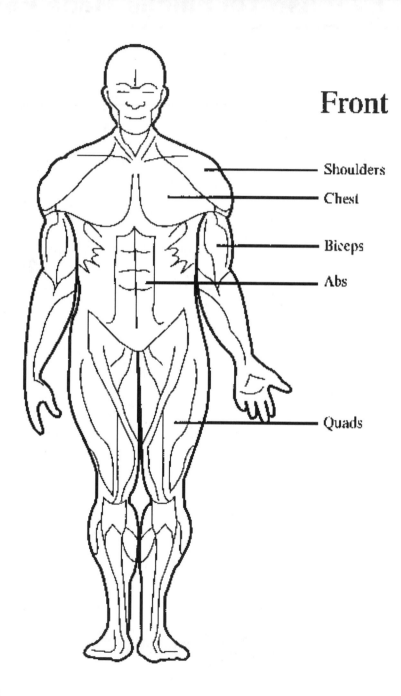

Front

Shoulders

Chest

Biceps

Abs

Quads

Basic Muscle Chart

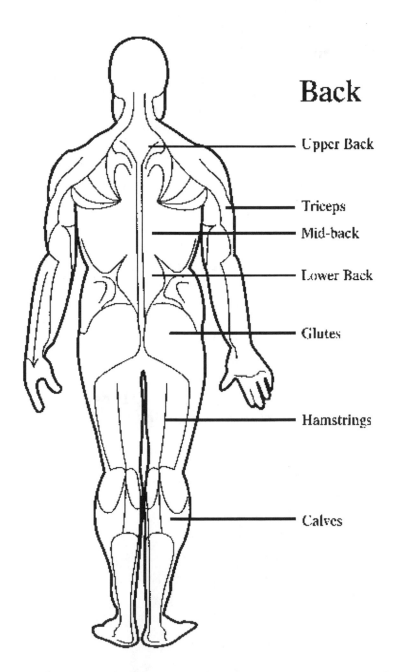

Back

Upper Back

Triceps

Mid-back

Lower Back

Glutes

Hamstrings

Calves

Legs

Leg Press

Target Muscles: Quads, Hamstrings, Glutes
Recommended Starting Weight: 50-100 lbs.

- Adjust the backrest so it is in the middle (higher up if you are small person, lower if you are larger).
- Back and buttocks firmly against the pads.
- Place your feet on top half of the platform.
- Feet shoulder width apart.
- Toes slightly pointed out about 10 degrees.
- Grasp handles, push up platform and unlock weights.
- Slowly lower knees towards your chest.
- When your legs go slightly past 90 degrees, (100-110 degrees) stop. Make sure your buttocks do not start to lift up. If it does, stop, you have gone too far. That can put undue stress on your back.
- Slowly push the weights up, through your heels. This will take pressure off your knees.
- Stop right before your knees lock out.
- Repeat until set is complete.
- **Tip: Find out how much the Leg Press weighs before you add weight. Every machine is different.**

Legs

Leg Press

❶

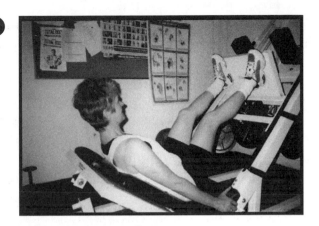

❷

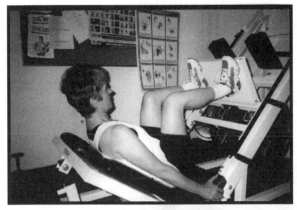

❸

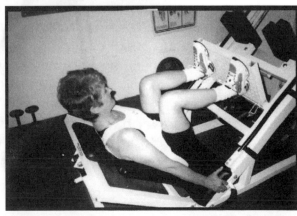

Legs

Barbell Squats

Target Muscles: Quads, Glutes, Hamstrings
Recommended Starting Weight: 25-50 lbs.

- **Tip: Use a squat rack or a spotter if available. If they are not available you should do Dumbbell Squats instead, until you feel more comfortable with weight training.**
- Place barbell on your upper back, not on your neck (use a bar pad if available).
- Feet shoulder width apart, toes slightly pointed out about 10 degrees.
- Focus eyes straight ahead during entire movement.
- Slowly lower, bending at the knees (think of sitting down in a chair).
- Your hips and buttocks go back. Knees straight over your feet.
- Knees behind your feet (if your knees are going in front of your feet too much, it puts undue stress on your knees. Make sure your rear end is going out).
- Keep your back straight (your back will be flat but will be about a 70-80 degree angle to the floor).
- Stop when your quads become parallel to the floor (this is your goal, but start by only lowering a short distance until you learn the exercise and become stronger).
- Push straight up under control.
- Breath out when you are half way up in the return phase.
- Stop right before your knees lock out.
- Repeat until set is complete.
- **Tip: If your lower back starts to develop a dull throb, stop and rest. Your lower back will probably be the first muscles to become tired, but will become stronger with practice.**

Barbell Squats

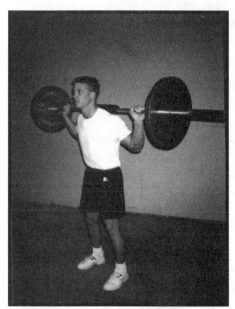

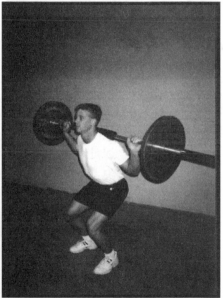

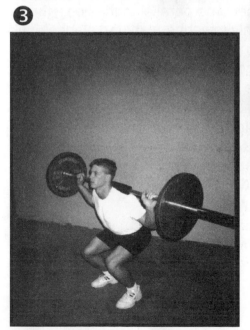

Legs

Dumbbell Squats

Target Muscles: Quads, Glutes, Hamstrings
Recommended Starting Weight: 5-15 lbs.

- Grasp dumbbells, palms facing each other at your sides.
- Feet shoulder width apart (or a little narrower so the dumbbells do not get in the way), toes slightly pointed out about 10 degrees.
- Focus eyes straight ahead during entire movement.
- Slowly lower, bending at the knees (think of sitting down in a chair).
- Your hips and buttocks go back. Knees straight over your feet.
- Knees behind your feet (if your knees are going in front of your feet too much, it puts undue stress on your knees. Make sure your rear end is going out).
- Keep your back straight (Your back will be flat but will be about a 70-80 degree angle to the floor).
- Stop when your quads become parallel to the floor (this is your goal, but start by only lowering a short distance until you learn the exercise and become stronger).
- Push straight up under control.
- Breath out when you are half way up in the return phase.
- Stop right before your knees lock out.
- Repeat until set is complete.
- **Tip: If your heels start to lift up while lowering, use small weight plates (5 or 10 lbs.) under your heels to help stabilize your body (see illustration).**

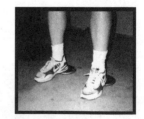

Dumbbell Squats

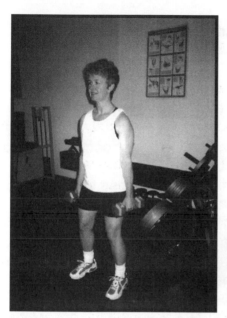

❶

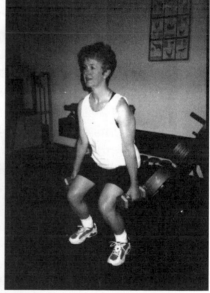

❷

❸

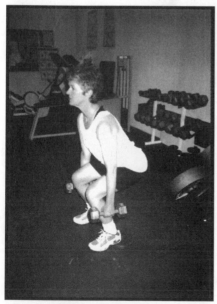

Legs

Lunges

Target Muscles: Hamstrings, Glutes, Quads
Recommended Starting Weight: 0

- You exercise one leg at a time.
- Grasp a bench, machine, etc. - something stable.
- Step forward with lead leg.
- Slowly lower straight down, keeping your back flat (do not lean forward).
- Bend knee of lead leg until it reaches close to 90 degree angle (in the beginning, only bend your front knee as far as you feel comfortable).
- Keep knee over and behind lead foot. Make sure you are going straight up and down. Do <u>not</u> lean forward.
- Knee of back leg should be a few inches off the floor.
- Push straight up.
- Stop right before your front knee locks out.
- Repeat until set is complete.
- Switch lead leg.
- **Tip: When you become stronger you can do lunges without holding on to a stable object. After that becomes too easy, you can add dumbbells in each hand for more resistance.**

Lunges

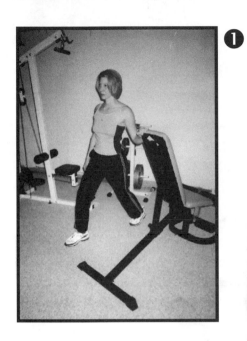

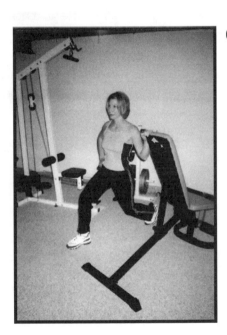

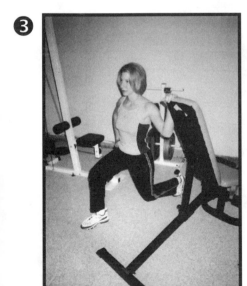

Legs

Leg Extensions

Target Muscles: Quads
Recommended Starting Weight: 20-40 lbs.

- Sit on the Leg Extension machine.
- Back firmly against the back pad.
- Back of knee against pad (adjust machine if needed).
- Lower leg pad on lower shin (adjust machine if needed).
- Slowly raise the weight until thigh is fully flexed and hold for a second, feeling your quads flex.
- Do not hyperextend knees by raising the weight to fast.
- Slowly lower.
- Stop before your lower leg goes past a 90 degree angle (by doing this, it keeps undue pressure off your knees).
- Repeat set until complete.

Legs

Leg Extensions

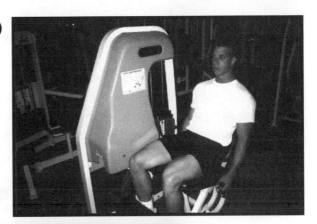

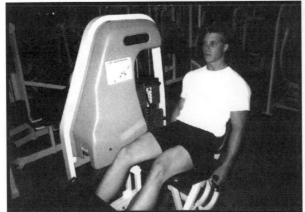

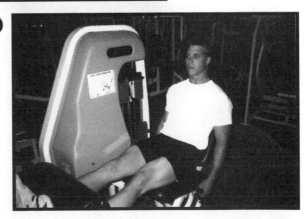

Legs

Leg Curls

Target Muscles: Hamstrings
Recommended Starting Weight: 20-40 lbs.

- Lie face down on the Leg Curl machine.
- Knees right behind the thigh pad.
- Lower leg pad above your heels.
- Grab handles or the bench.
- Pull the weight up slowly, especially the first 2-3 inches (this will emphasize the hamstrings).
- Stop when your feet are straight up or close to your rear end.
- Keep your hips in contact with the bench at all times.
- Slowly lower the weight.
- Stop right before your knees lock out.
- Repeat until set is complete.

Leg Curls

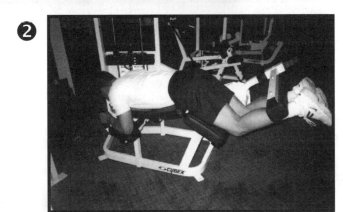

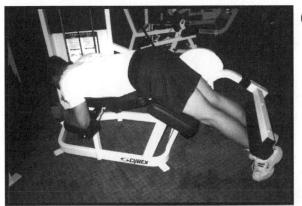

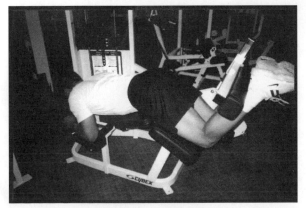

Legs

Deadlifts

Target Muscles: Hamstrings, Glutes, Lower Back
Recommended Starting Weight: 0-45 lbs.

- Grasp barbell, palms facing you.
- Hands shoulder width apart.
- Feet straight-ahead, about a foot apart.
- Hold barbell with arms straight, at mid thigh.
- Keep back flat, shoulders back, chest out and knees slightly bent throughout movement.
- Lower bar, right in front of your body, until about mid-shin level (do not go too far down, only until it feels comfortable).
- Hips and rear end go back, bending at the waist.
- Feel a stretch in your hamstrings.
- Pull up to starting position, concentrating on your hamstrings, not your back.
- Repeat until set is complete.
- **Tip: Remember to keep your back flat. Do not round your back. Keep your head in the neutral position.**
- **Tip: Do not use too heavy of weights.**

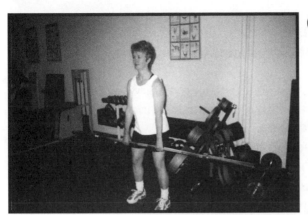

❶

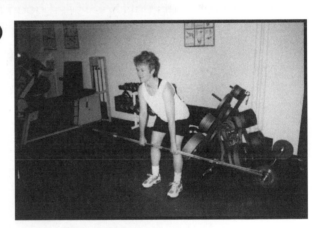

❷

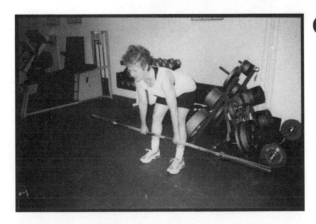

❸

Legs

Calf Raises

Target Muscles: Calf
Recommended Starting Weight: 50-100 lbs.

- Do calf raises on the Leg Press machine. If it is not available, you can use a calf block, various calf machines, or the stairs.
- Place balls of feet on the edge of the platform, knees relatively straight.
- Push up as far as possible until you feel a stretch at the top of the movement.
- Slowly lower heels until you feel a good stretch in your calves.
- Repeat until set is complete.

Calf Raises

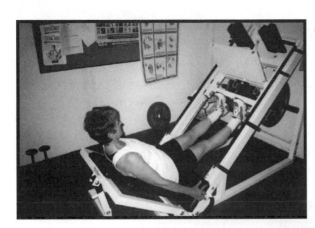

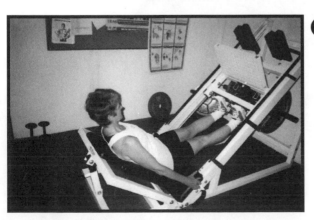

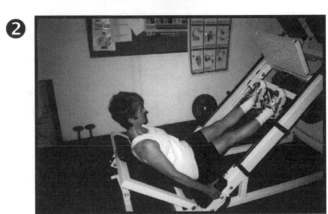

Abs

Crunches

Target Muscles: Abs
Recommended Starting Weight: 0

- Lie on your back.
- Knees bent, feet on the floor.
- Put hands across your chest, do not put your hands behind your head.
- Curl up about 30-degrees (do not go up all the way).
- Hold for a second.
- Slowly lower until right before your shoulders fully touch the floor (it keeps tension on your abs).
- Repeat until set is complete.
- **Tip: Keep your stomach flexed during the entire exercise,** *" like you are getting ready for someone to punch you in the stomach."*
- **Tip: When adding weight for resistance, hold a weight plate across your chest.**

Crunches

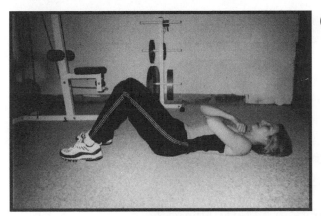

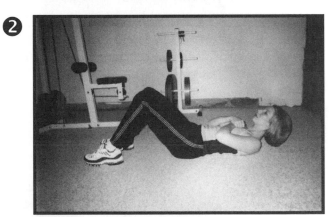

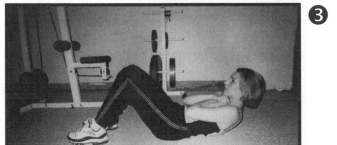

Abs

Ab Bench Crunches

Target Muscles: Abs
Recommended Starting Weight: 0

- Set bench to approximately 10-30 degree decline.
- Lock-in legs.
- Place hands across chest.
- Do not put your hands behind your head, you can pull on your neck and spine.
- Slowly lower your body, keeping your back slightly rounded.
- Lower upper body until nearing parallel to the floor (do not go too low until you are strong enough!).
- Keep abs tight throughout movement.
- Return to starting position, stopping just before you are straight up to keep tension on the abs.
- Repeat until set is complete

Abs

Ab Bench Crunches

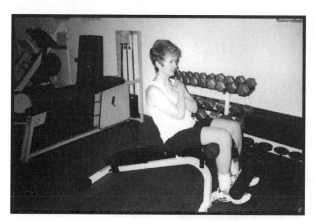

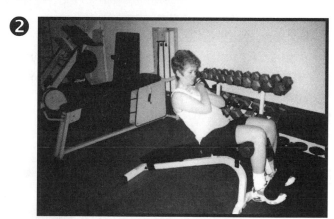

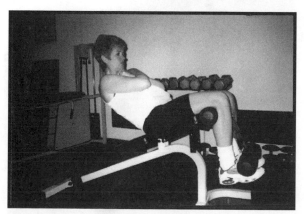

Abs

Reverse Crunches

Target Muscles: Lower Abs
Recommended Starting Weight: 0

- Set bench at approximately a 30-degree decline.
- Lay on your back, head at the top of the bench (make sure your head is flat on the bench).
- Hang on to the top of the bench (this is the hardest part of the exercise for some people, just grab onto whatever you can, it will become easier).
- Curl up your legs as far as you feel comfortable, knees bent.
- Pause for a second at the top.
- Slowly lower legs.
- Lower as far as you feel comfortable (your lower back and abs will become stronger quickly with this exercise).
- Repeat until set is complete.
- **Tip: Use a spotter to help lift your legs.**
- **Tip: If your lower back is weak, substitute another ab exercise until you feel stronger.**

Reverse Crunches

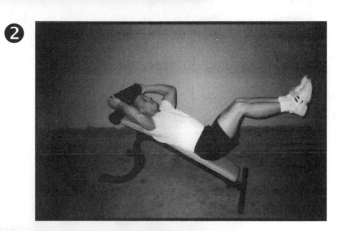

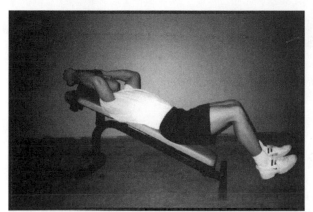

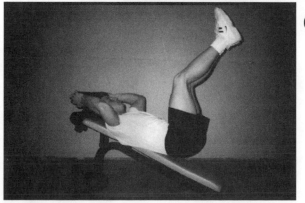

Chest

Barbell Bench Press

Target Muscles: Chest, Shoulders, Triceps
Recommended Starting Weight: 20-45 lbs.

- Lay flat on the bench with your feet on the floor or bench, keeping your lower back flat.
- Grasp barbell, palms facing forward, slightly wider than shoulder width apart (you can experiment with your hand position but do not go too wide or narrow because this can put undue stress on your shoulders).
- Slowly lower the bar to your mid-chest with elbows straight out to the sides.
- Lightly touch middle of the chest (do not bounce). Upper and lower arms should be at about a right angle.
- Feel a stretch in your chest and mentally push with your chest muscles.
- Stop right before you lock out on top.
- Repeat until set is complete.
- **Tip: Make sure to use a spotter.**

Chest

Barbell Bench Press

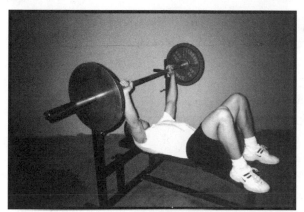

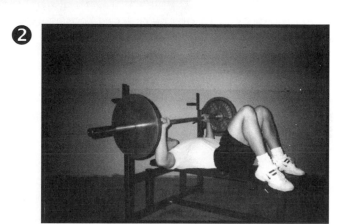

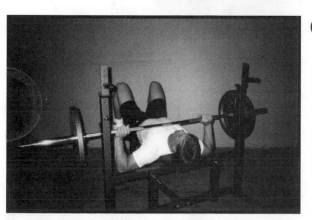

Chest

Dumbbell Bench Press

Target Muscles: Chest, Shoulders, Triceps
Recommended Starting Weight: 5-15 lbs.

- Lay flat on the bench with your feet on the floor or bench, keeping your lower back flat.
- Bring dumbbells to the starting position with your palms facing forward towards your feet.
- Slowly lower dumbbells, elbows straight out to the sides.
- Lower until you feel a good stretch in your chest and your arms are at about a 90-degree angle (if your front shoulders start to pull too much, stop. You will become stronger and more flexible with practice).
- Push straight up.
- Stop right before you lock out on top.
- Repeat until set is complete.

Dumbbell Bench Press

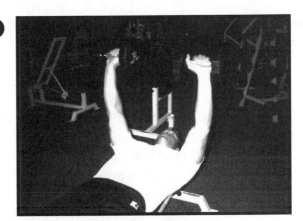

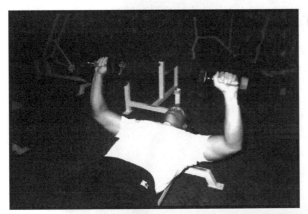

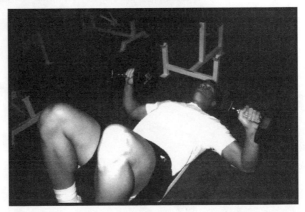

Chest

Incline Dumbbell Bench Press

Target Muscles: Upper Chest, Shoulders, Triceps
Recommended Starting Weight: 5-15 lbs.

- Set or use a bench with approximately a 45-degree incline.
- Feet on floor and lower back pushed against the backrest.
- Bring dumbbells to the starting position with your palms facing forward towards your feet.
- Slowly lower dumbbells, elbows straight out to the sides.
- Lower until you feel a good stretch in your upper chest and your arms are at about a 90-degree angle (if your front shoulders start to pull too much, stop. You will become stronger and more flexible with practice).
- Push straight up.
- Stop right before your elbows lock out on top.
- Repeat until set is complete.

Incline Dumbbell Bench Press

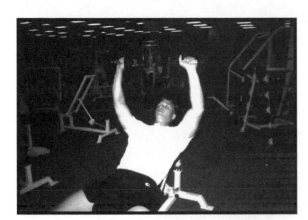

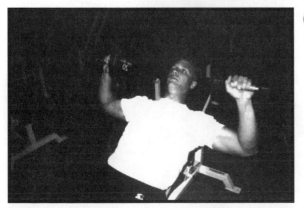

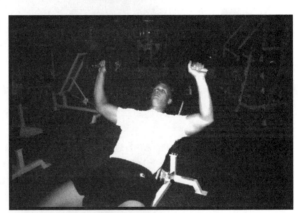

Chest

Dumbbell Flys

Target Muscles: Chest
Recommended Starting Weight: 3-10 lbs.

- Lie on bench, feet on the floor or bench.
- Bring the dumbbells to the starting position.
- Palms facing each other.
- Keep elbows slightly bent during the movement.
- Slowly lower dumbbells straight out to your sides.
- Keep chest muscles tight when slowly lowering the dumbbells.
- Lower until you feel a stretch in your chest muscles.
- Make sure you stop lowering if you start to feel your front shoulders pulling too much.
- Mentally pull up with your chest, not concentrating on your arms.
- Keep chest flexed throughout movement (especially the top part of the exercise).
- Repeat until set is complete.
- **Tip: The movement should be in an arc, with gravity pulling the dumbbells down (keep your arms about the same angle throughout the movement, this is not a pressing movement).**

Chest

Dumbbell Flys

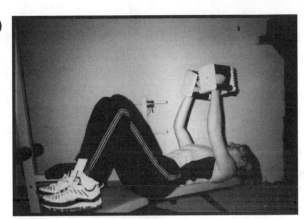

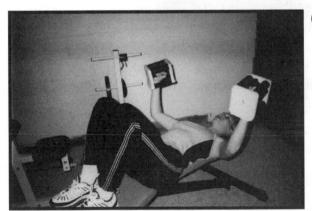

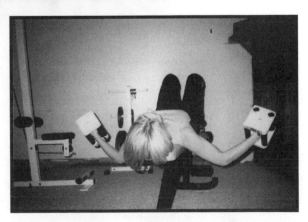

Shoulders

Barbell Shoulder Press

Target Muscles: Shoulders, Triceps
Recommended Starting Weight: 10-30 lbs.

- Stand with feet shoulder width apart.
- Keep knees slightly bent.
- Bring barbell to the starting position.
- Palms forward, just slightly wider than shoulder width apart.
- Push barbell straight up in front of your face (be sure to look straight ahead during entire movement, this will keep your back as straight as possible).
- Stop right before elbows lock out.
- Slowly lower barbell to <u>chin level</u> (keeps tension on your shoulders).
- Repeat until set is complete.
- **Tip: Use a spotter if available.**

Shoulders

Barbell Shoulder Press

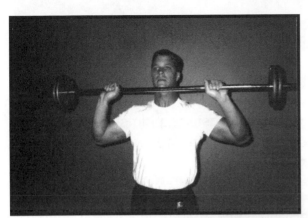

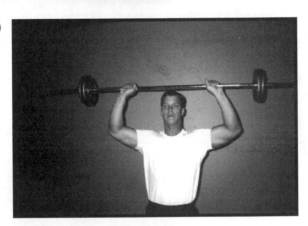

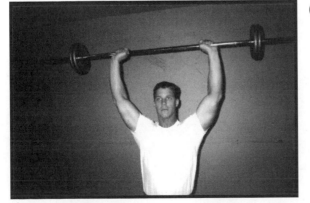

Shoulders

Dumbbell Shoulder Press

Target Muscles: Shoulders, Triceps
Recommended Starting Weight: 3-10 lbs.

- Seated, back flat against bench, feet firmly on the floor.
- Grasp dumbbells.
- Bring dumbbells to starting position, palms facing forward.
- Arms should be at a right angle.
- Push straight up, stopping right before your elbows lock out.
- Make sure to keep your back straight (keep it pressed against the backrest).
- Slowly lower.
- Stop when dumbbells are in line with your ears, arms at a right angle (it keeps tension on your shoulders).
- Repeat until set is complete.

Dumbbell Shoulder Press

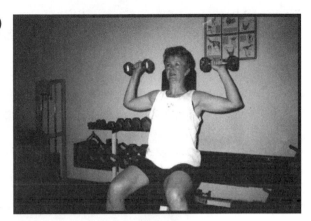

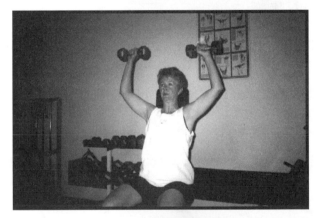

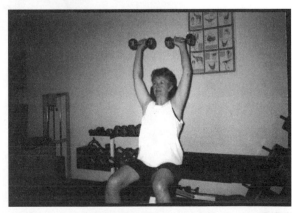

Shoulders

Side Lateral Raises

Target Muscles: Shoulders
Recommended Starting Weight: 1-8 lbs.

- Standing.
- Dumbbells at your sides and palms facing each other.
- Keep elbows bent during the entire movement (you will need to concentrate on this).
- Raise the dumbbells out to the sides (like you are flying).
- Stop when the dumbbells are in line with or slightly above your head.
- Slowly lower, keeping elbows bent.
- Repeat until set is complete.

Shoulders

Side Lateral Raises

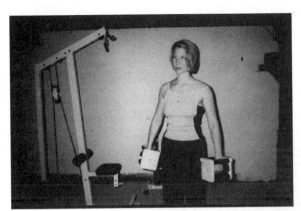

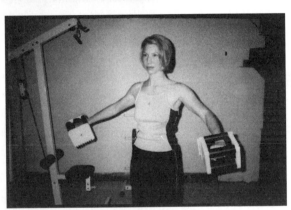

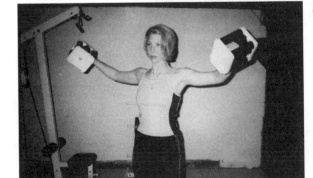

Back

Lat Pulldown (wide grip)

Target Muscles: Upper & Mid Back, Biceps
Recommended Starting Weight: 30-60 lbs.

- Grasp the straight bar with an overhand grip, palms facing away from you.
- Hands 2-3 inches wider than your shoulders (do not go too wide, this can put undue stress on your shoulders).
- Holding bar, sit down and lock knees under pad (adjust height of pad if needed).
- Lean back, with chest out during entire movement.
- First movement should be pulling your shoulder blades back and together (think of someone putting a finger between your shoulder blades and you trying to squeeze their finger).
- Pull the bar all the way down to the mid-upper chest area, concentrating on your upper back.
- Elbows half way between your sides and straight out.
- Stop for a second, then slowly resist the bar all the way up (remember to keep your chest out and shoulders back through the entire movement).
- Keep back muscles tight.
- Return the bar all the way up until you feel a slight stretch in your mid/upper back muscles.
- Repeat until set is complete.

Lat Pulldown (wide grip)

 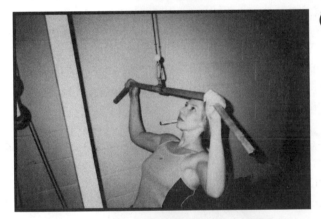

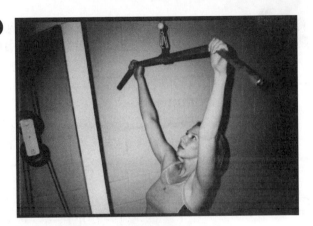

 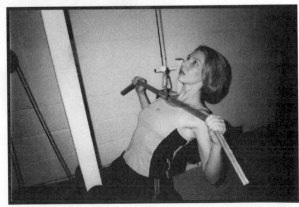

Back

Lat Pulldown (Underhand)

Target Muscles: Mid Back, Biceps
Recommended Starting Weight: 30-60 lbs.

Same as Lat Pulldown (wide grip) except:
- Underhand grip with palms facing you.
- Hands approximately 1 –2 feet apart.
- Pull to low-mid chest area.
- Elbows along the sides of your body.

Lat Pulldown (Underhand)

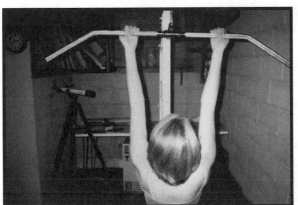

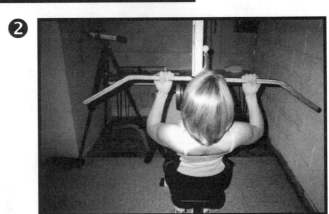

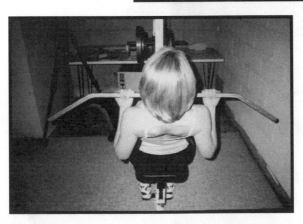

Back

Lat Pulldown (triangle bar)

Target Muscles: Mid-outer Back, Biceps
Recommended Starting Weight: 30-60 lbs.

Same as Lat Pulldown (wide grip) except:
- Use the triangle bar (also called the V-Bar).
- Palms facing each other.
- Pull to mid-chest.
- Elbows along the sides of your body.
- Concentrate on mid and outer sides of back.

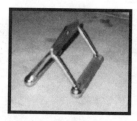

Triangle Bar

Back

Lat Pulldown (Triangle Bar)

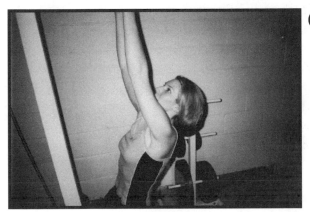

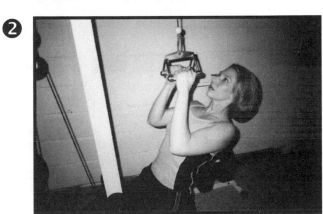

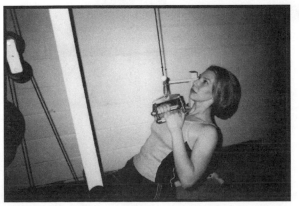

Back

Dumbbell Pullovers

Target Muscles: Back, Triceps, Chest
Recommended Starting Weight: 10-20 lbs.

- Lay on the bench with your feet on the floor or bench.
- Your head at the end of the bench (make sure your head is supported on the bench).
- Grasp a dumbbell on the inside end with your palms flat, overlapping each other securely (see illustration below).
- Keep elbows in and pointed forward, towards your feet.
- Slowly lower the dumbbell behind your head (be careful not to hit your head!).
- Keep your muscles tight!
- Lower until upper arms are beside your head and lower arms are bent.
- Feel a good stretch in your abs, back and triceps (do not go too far down right away. If your shoulders start to feel weak, stop. You will become stronger and more flexible with practice).
- Slowly pull up with your elbows, not your hands. This will emphasize your back muscles.
- Straighten your arms towards the top of movement.
- Stop when the dumbbell is straight over your chest-shoulder area.
- Repeat until set is complete.

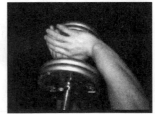

Dumbbell Pullovers

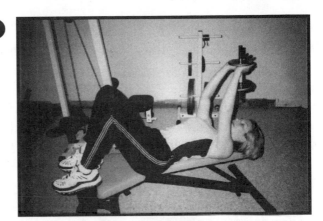

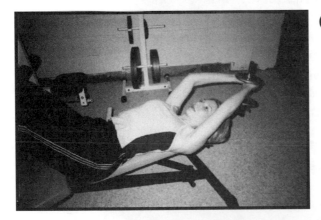

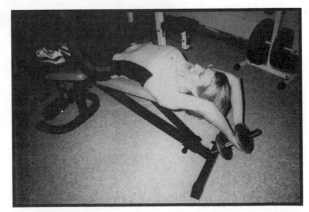

Back

Dumbbell Rows

Target Muscles: Back, Biceps
Recommended Starting Weight: 10-20 lbs.

- You exercise one arm at a time.
- Exercising your right arm.
- On a flat bench place your left knee and left hand.
- Space your knee and hand far enough apart so your back is straight, not rounded.
- Keep your left elbow slightly bent throughout the movement so you do not bend it backwards.
- Place your right foot towards the back of the bench (on the floor), so your leg is out of the way.
- Grasp the dumbbell with palm facing you.
- Pull the dumbbell up as far as possible like you are starting a lawnmower (the first movement should be pulling your right shoulder back and then pulling through with your arm).
- Keep elbow along side of your body.
- During the movement slightly turn your body up so you can lift the weight higher.
- Pause at the top and try to feel your mid-outer back muscles doing the work (remember to keep your left elbow slightly bent the whole time).
- Slowly lower the dumbbell, turning your body back towards the floor.
- Lower until you get a slight stretch in your middle back.
- Repeat until set is complete.
- Repeat exercise with your left arm.

Dumbbell Rows

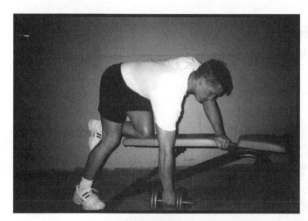

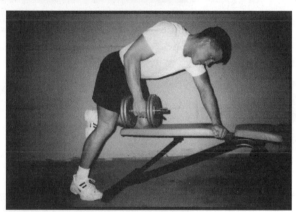

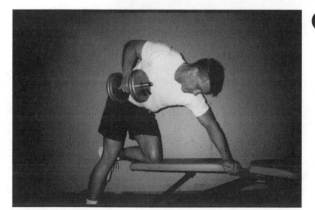

Biceps

Barbell Curls

Target Muscles: Biceps
Recommended Starting Weight: 10-25 lbs.

- Standing, feet shoulder width apart.
- Knees slightly bent.
- Palms forward, slightly wider than shoulder width apart.
- Elbows touching your sides.
- Curl the weight up towards your shoulders/chin area until biceps are fully contracted.
- Look straight ahead and do not to arch your back during lifting phase.
- Slowly lower the weight.
- Stop right before your elbows lock out.
- Repeat until set is complete.

Biceps

Barbell Curls

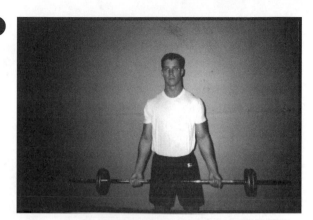

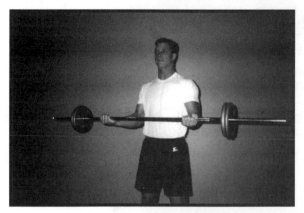

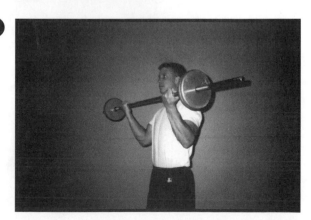

Biceps

Dumbbell Curls

Target Muscles: Biceps
Recommended Starting Weight: 5-15 lbs.

- Seated, feet firmly on the floor.
- Back straight.
- Dumbbells hanging at your sides.
- Palms facing each other.
- Elbows pressed against your sides (elbows do not move).
- Curl dumbbells at the same time towards your shoulders, rotating palms so they are facing up when biceps are fully contracted.
- Slowly lower weight, rotating palms back so they are facing each other again at the bottom.
- Stop right before elbows lock out.
- Repeat until set is complete.

Dumbbell Curls

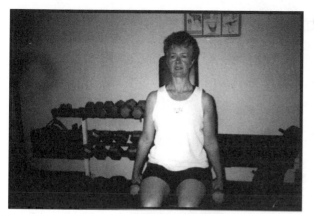

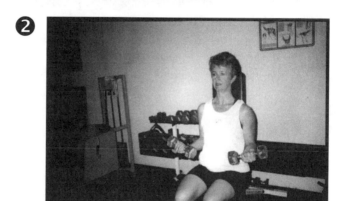

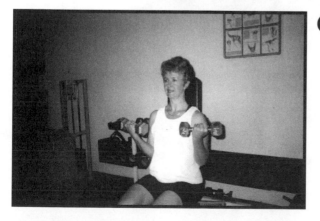

Triceps

Tricep Pushdowns

Target Muscles: Triceps
Recommended Starting Weight: 15-30 lbs.

- Stand, facing the pull down machine, about a foot away.
- Keep your back straight, knees slightly bent and feet shoulder width apart.
- Grasp bar, palms facing down, about a foot apart.
- Pull the bar down so your elbows are touching your sides. Then your elbows will not move during the exercise.
- Push straight down until arms are straight (you should feel your triceps contract).
- Slowly resist weight until about chest height. (Remember your elbows do not move).
- Repeat until set is complete.

Tricep Pushdowns

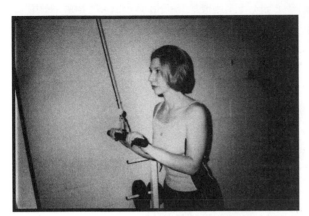

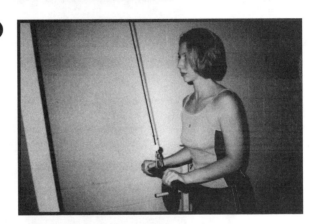

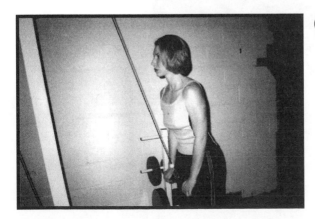

Models

Thanks to Scott, Dusty and Marianne. They are actual clients who lift weights 1-3 times per week using *Weight Training Workouts that Work* with fantastic results!

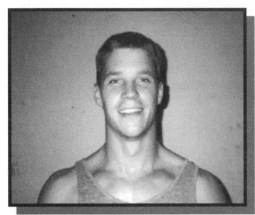

Scott Jensen

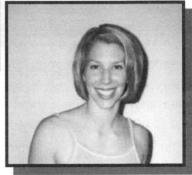

Dusty Rafter

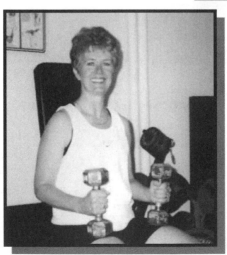

Marianne Breitbach

Afterword

You have learned a new set of skills that will keep you fit and healthy for the rest of you life! What can be better than that? Weight training is a very important part of millions of peoples' lives. It is the best way to keep fit and to improve your body year after year. It is the fountain of youth!

Best of luck,

James Orvis

Questions about Weight Training Workouts that Work?

james@weighttrainingworkouts.com

Need more copies? New workouts? Volume II?
Order online – always free shipping and lowest prices!

www.weighttrainingworkouts.com

About the Author

James Orvis is a certified personal trainer. Training in private residences, health clubs and corporate settings he has developed a simple method for maximum results. Working with hundreds of men and women of all ages, he has discovered what people need – easy to follow, proven weight training workouts that keep you fit, firm and healthy. He lives in Minnesota with his wife, Traci.

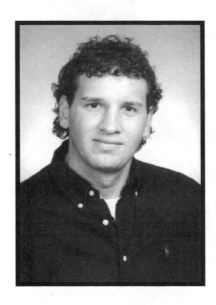